HOW TO HEALTHIER AND RIGHT

Unique guide To Losing Weight The Healthy Way

Vanessa D Daniel

TABLE OF CONTENT

Chapter 2..2

Chapter 3 2
Chapter 4 2
Chapter 1 1

Chapter 1

Eating Right
The fundamentals of healthy eating

While a few outrageous eating regimens might be recommended in any case, we as a whole need an equilibrium of protein, fat, sugars, fiber, nutrients, and minerals in our eating regimens to support a sound body. You don't have to wipe out specific classes of food from your eating regimen, but instead, select the best choices from every classification.

Protein gives you the energy to get moving and continue onward while additionally supporting your mindset and mental capability. An excess of protein can be hurtful to individuals with kidney illness, however, the most recent exploration recommends that large numbers of us need all the more great protein, particularly as we age. That doesn't mean you need to eat more creature items; an assortment of plant-based wellsprings of protein every day can guarantee your body gets all the fundamental protein it needs.

Fat. Not all fat is something similar. While awful fats can wreck your eating routine and increment your gamble of specific illnesses, great fats safeguard your mind and heart. Solid fats like omega-3s are imperative to your physical and close-to-home well-being. Remembering more solid fat for your eating routine can assist with working on your state of mind, help your prosperity, and, surprisingly, trim your waistline.

Fiber. Eating food sources high in dietary fiber (grains, organic products, vegetables, nuts, and beans) can assist you with remaining ordinary and lower your gamble of coronary illness, stroke, and diabetes. It can likewise work on your skin and even assist you with getting more fit.

Calcium. As well as prompting osteoporosis, not getting sufficient calcium in your eating routine can likewise add to tension, sadness, and rest challenges. Whatever your age or orientation, it's crucial to remember calcium-rich food varieties for your eating routine, limit those that exhaust calcium, and get sufficient magnesium and nutrients D and K to assist calcium with taking care of its business.

Starches are one of your body's principal wellsprings of energy. Yet, most ought to come from perplexing, crude carbs (vegetables, entire grains, organic products) as opposed to sugars and refined carbs. Scaling back white bread, cakes, starches, and sugar can forestall quick spikes in glucose, changes in mindset and energy, and the development of fat, particularly around your waistline.

Doing the change to a solid eating regimen

Changing to a solid eating regimen doesn't need to be a go big or go home suggestion. You don't need to be awesome, you don't need to take out food sources you appreciate, and you don't need to change everything at the same time that generally just prompts cheating or abandoning your new eating plan.

A superior methodology is to make a couple of little changes all at once. Keeping your objectives unobtrusive can assist you with accomplishing more in the long haul without feeling denied or overpowered by a significant eating routine update. Consider arranging a solid eating routine with various little, reasonable advances like adding a serving of mixed greens to your eating routine one time each day.

As your little improvement becomes propensity, you can keep on adding more solid decisions.To place yourself in a good position, attempt to keep things basic. Eating a better eating regimen doesn't need to be confused. Rather than being excessively worried about counting calories, for instance, consider your eating regimen concerning variety, assortment, and newness. Center around staying away from bundled and handled food varieties and picking all the more new fixings whenever the situation allows. Plan your very own greater amount of feasts. Preparing more dinners at home can assist you with assuming responsibility for what you're eating and better screen precisely everything that goes into your food. You'll eat fewer calories and stay away from the substance-added substances, added sugar, and unfortunate facts of bundled and takeout food varieties that can leave you feeling tired, swollen, and peevish, and worsen side effects of despondency, stress, and tension.

Roll out the right improvements. While scaling back undesirable food sources in your eating routine, supplanting them with sound alternatives is significant. Supplanting hazardous trans fats with sound fats (like exchanging seared chicken for barbecued salmon) will have a constructive outcome on your well-being. Exchanging creature fats for refined starches, however (like exchanging your morning meal bacon for a doughnut), won't bring down your gamble for coronary illness or work on your state of mind.

Peruse the marks. It's vital to know about what's in your food as makers frequently conceal a lot of sugar or undesirable fats in bundled food, even food professing to be sound.

Center around how you feel after eating. This will assist with encouraging solid new propensities and tastes. The better the food you eat, the better you'll feel after a feast. The more low-quality food you eat, the almost certain you are to feel awkward, sick, or depleted of energy.

Drink a lot of water. Water helps flush our frameworks of side effects and poisons, yet a large number of us carry on with life dried out causing sluggishness, low energy, and migraines. It's generally expected to confuse thirst with hunger, so remaining very much hydrated will likewise assist you with pursuing better food decisions.

Balance: essential to any solid eating routine

What is the balance? It implies eating just as the need might arise. You ought to feel fulfilled toward the finish of a feast, yet at the same time not stuffed. For the vast majority of us, balance implies eating short of what we do now. However, it doesn't mean taking out the food varieties you love.

Having bacon for breakfast one time per week, for instance, could be viewed as balanced on the off chance that you follow it with a solid lunch and supper – however not assuming you follow it with a crate of doughnuts and a wiener pizza.

Make an effort not to consider specific food sources "beyond reach." When you boycott specific food varieties, it's normal to need those food sources more, and afterward, feel like a disappointment on the off chance that you yield to enticement. Begin by decreasing part sizes of unfortunate food sources and not eating them as frequently. As you decrease your admission of unfortunate food sources, you might end up needing them less or considering them just periodic guilty pleasures.

Think more modest segments. Serving sizes have expanded as of late. While feasting out, pick a starter rather than a course, split a dish with a companion, and don't organize anything. At home, obvious prompts can assist with segment sizes. Your serving of meat, fish, or chicken ought to be the size of a deck of cards and a portion of a cup of mashed potato, rice, or pasta is about the size of a customary light.

By serving your dinners on more modest plates or in bowls, you can fool your cerebrum into believing it's a bigger part. On the off chance that you don't feel fulfilled toward the finish of a dinner, add more salad greens or adjust the feast with a natural product.

Take as much time as necessary. It's essential to dial back and consider food sustenance as opposed to only something to swallow in the middle between gatherings or while heading to get the children. It requires a couple of moments for your cerebrum to let your body know that it has had sufficient food, so eat gradually and quit eating before you feel full.

Eat with others whenever the situation allows. Eating alone, particularly before the TV or PC, frequently prompts careless gorging.Limit nibble food sources in the home. Be cautious about the food sources you keep within reach. It's more difficult to eat with some restraint assuming that you have undesirable tidbits and treats good to go. All things considered, encircle yourself with solid decisions and when you're prepared to compensate yourself with a unique treat, go out and get it then.

Control close-to-home eating. We don't necessarily in every case eat just to fulfill hunger. A large number of us likewise go to food to ease pressure or adapt to undesirable feelings like bitterness, forlornness, or weariness. Be that as it may, by learning better ways of overseeing pressure and feelings, you can recover command over the food you eat and your sentiments.

Add more leafy foods to your eating regimen

Leafy foods are low in calories and supplements thick, and that implies they are loaded with nutrients, minerals, cell reinforcements, and fiber. Center around eating the suggested everyday measure of no less than five servings of products of the soil and it will normally top you off and assist you with scaling back unfortunate food sources. A serving is a portion of a cup of crude natural product or veg or a little apple or banana, for instance. A large portion of us needs to twofold the sum we now eat. To increment your admission:Add cancer prevention agent-rich berries to your number one breakfast cereal.Eat a mixture of sweet natural products oranges, mangos, pineapple, grapes for dessert.Trade your typical rice or pasta side dish for a vivid plate of mixed greens.Rather than eating handled nibble food sources, nibble on vegetables like carrots, snow peas, or cherry tomatoes alongside a zesty hummus plunge or peanut butter.

The most effective method to make vegetables delicious while plain plates of mixed greens and steamed veggies can immediately become dull, there are a lot of ways of adding taste to your vegetable dishes.Add tone. Not in the least do more splendid, more profound shaded vegetables contain higher centralizations of nutrients, minerals, and cell reinforcements, however, they can fluctuate the flavor and make dinners all the more outwardly engaging. Add variety utilizing new or sundried tomatoes, coated carrots or beets, cooked red cabbage wedges, yellow squash, or sweet, bright peppers.

Spice up salad greens. Branch out past lettuce. Kale, arugula, spinach, mustard greens, broccoli, and Chinese cabbage are undeniably loaded with supplements. To add flavor to your serving of mixed greens, have a go at showering with olive oil, adding a fiery dressing, or sprinkling with almond cuts, chickpeas, a little bacon, parmesan, or goat cheddar.

Fulfill your sweet tooth. Normally sweet vegetables —, for example, carrots, beets, yams, sweet potatoes, onions, ringer peppers, and squash — add pleasantness to your dinners and diminish your desire for added sugar. Add them to soups, stews, or pasta sauces for a delightful sweet kick.

Cook green beans, broccoli, Brussels fledglings, and asparagus in new ways. Rather than bubbling or steaming these solid sides, take a stab at barbecuing, cooking, or searing them with stew chips, garlic, shallots, mushrooms, or onion. Or then again marinate in tart lemon or lime before cooking.

Chapter 2

Being In Charge Of What You Eat

What we eat affects how we feel. Food should make us feel good. It tastes great and nourishes our bodies. If you eat too little or eat too much, however, your health and quality of life could be affected. This can result in negative feelings toward food.

By learning how to make healthier and more mindful choices, you may be able to control compulsive eating, binging, and weight gain. By taking charge of your appetite, you may also gain a feeling of calm, high energy levels, and alertness from the foods you eat.

Overall, there are many benefits to changing deep-seated, unhealthy eating habits, such as:

An increase in energy level and alertness.

A more positive relationship with food.

Improved health.

Easier movement.

What role does psychology play in weight management?

Psychology is the science of behavior. It is the study of how and why people do what they do. For people trying to manage their weight, psychology addresses:

Behavior: Treatment involves identifying the person’s eating patterns and finding ways to change eating behaviors.

Cognition (thinking): Therapy focuses on identifying self-defeating thinking patterns that contribute to weight management problems.

What treatments are used for weight management?

Cognitive behavioral treatment is the approach most often used because it deals with both thinking patterns and behavior. Some areas that are addressed through cognitive behavioral treatment include:

Determining the person's "readiness for change": This involves an awareness of what needs to be done to achieve your goals and then committing to doing it.

Learning how to self-monitor: Self-monitoring helps you become more aware of what triggers you to eat at the moment and more mindful of your food choices and portions. It also helps you stay focused on achieving long-term progress.

Breaking linkages: The focus here is on stimulus control, such as not eating in particular settings, and not keeping unhealthy food choices in your home. Cognitive behavioral treatment also teaches distraction replacing eating with healthier alternatives as a skill for coping with stress.

Cognitive therapy addresses how you think about food. It helps you recognize self-defeating patterns of thinking that can undermine your success at eating healthier and managing your weight/weight loss. It also helps you learn and practice using positive coping self-statements.

Examples of self-defeating thoughts include:

"This is too hard. I can't do it."

"If I don't make it to my target weight, I've failed."

"Now that I've lost weight, I can go back to eating any way I want."

Examples of positive coping self-statements include:
"I realize that I am overeating. I need to think about how I can stop this pattern of behavior."
"I need to understand what triggered my overeating, so I can create a plan to cope with it if I encounter the trigger again."
"Am I really hungry or is this just a craving? I will wait to see if this feeling passes."
What strategies will help me manage my weight?
To lose weight, it's helpful to change your thinking. Weight management is about making a lifestyle change. It's not going to happen if you rely on the short-term diet after a diet to lose weight.
To be successful, be aware of the role that eating plays in your life, and learn how to use positive thinking and behavioral coping strategies to manage your eating and your weight. To help get you started, here are a few tips:
Tips for healthy eating
Don't skip meals.

Do plan meals and snacks ahead of time.
Do keep track of your eating habits
Does limit night eating?
Do drink plenty of water.
Many people say that adopting diets low in salt, fat, sugar, or animal products alters their food preferences, and there's some scientific evidence to support this experience. Researchers have also investigated methods of modifying one's food preferences so more healthful foods will be more appealing. In general and not unexpectedly, flavor and food preferences are more malleable when we're young (indeed, in utero), but as adults, we can still work on them.
Several studies have shown that people who manage to follow a low-sodium diet for several months wind up preferring lower concentrations of salt in their food
Appetites for sugar and fat can also be changed, although

there's less experimental evidence for it. British researchers reported results in 2011 from a small study that showed that tastes changed to liking sweeter things after a month of drinking a sweetened energy drink.

How to avoid overeating

One expert on nutrition and behavior change has developed some behavioral techniques for reducing the ingestion of unhealthy calories. Brian Wansink, a Cornell professor and author of Mindless Eating, has identified five situations where people are particularly at risk for ingesting large quantities. He has called them "meal stuffing," "snack grazing," "restaurant indulging," "party binging," and "desktop or dashboard dining."

Vegetables contain bitter compounds — and some people have a genetic propensity to experience more bitterness from vegetables (as well as other foods) than other people do. Heightened bitterness can also obscure sweetness. Vegetables tend to be more palatable to more people when the bitter and sweet tastes are nicely balanced and form that complicated bittersweet experience.

If you keep an open mind and try a variety of vegetables, you might find varieties that contain bitter compounds to which you are less sensitive. You may respond more to the bitter compounds in, say, broccoli than those in kale.

Developing a taste for whole grains

According to dietary guidelines, at least half of the grain-based food we eat should be made from whole grains (and that is setting the bar too low). Most Americans don't even come close to meeting that recommendation, partly because whole grains tend to have a slightly more bitter taste and rougher texture than foods made with refined grains (think white bread).

One system for making entire grains more engaging is basically to blend in a few refined grains. You can do this at home by subbing around 50% of the flour in treat, biscuit, or bread recipes with entire wheat flour. Blending raw grain into meatballs, meatloaf, or burgers or adding grain, an entire grain that is gentle in flavor, as a thickener in soups and stews are other simple methods for slipping all the more entire grains into your eating regimen.

Yield to your longing a bit

Weight reduction and different sorts of diets have a long history of poor long-haul achievement. One potential clarification — among numerous — is that barring specific food varieties, and their flavors, stirs up our cravings for them. Yet again control is really smart.Exorbitant dietary limitations can prompt gorging. In one examination, female health food nuts and non-dieters were served either nothing, one milkshake, or two. Then, at that point, they were approached to taste and rate some frozen yogurt. Calorie counters who felt they had broken their eating regimens answered by indulging the frozen yogurt, whether or not they'd had a couple of milkshakes. The nondieters did nothing of the sort.

Chapter 3

The Link Between Eating Right and Exercising

Smart dieting and standard activity remain inseparable toward carrying on with a cheerful and useful life. One without the other is inadequate, making it critical to figure out some kind of harmony between the two. The connection between good dieting and normal activity is significant for some reasons. There is an obvious connection between food and exercise.

Without normal activity, good dieting isn't as advantageous

as well as the other way around. The two work together to keep you in great shape genuinely and intellectually. At the point when you accomplish this sort of equilibrium, you will probably have a more joyful and more useful life.

The greatest advantage of a sound dynamic way of life is to remember a general increment of your energy and a positive mindset. The best mix of diet and exercise sets you feeling better, yet it likewise makes you more mindful of your environmental elements. Without good food sources, you will not have the option to keep up with legitimate physical or psychological well-being.

While clearness comes from eating a sound eating routine, standard activity is the most effective way to keep your state of mind positive. At the point when you work out, it animates the synthetics in your cerebrum and you will naturally start to feel more joyful with your life.

The proverb monotony wears on the soul firmly connected with your general wellbeing. By taking part in a solid eating routine as well as exercise, you free yourself up to open doors you probably wouldn't have in any case. Good dieting makes the way for appreciating getting ready dinners at home with your friends and family and in any event, visiting neighborhood rancher's business sectors. As far as exercise, you can

help by taking part in exercises with your loved ones that keep you dynamic and continually moving. Food gives energy.Practice consumes energy.

Yet, practicing just to "consume" the calories you devour can cause it to feel like there is an immediate exchange occurring between the food sources you eat and your exercises. This outlook could make you believe that the solution to weight reduction is eating less, preparing more, or both.

This value-based speculation can be hazardous for various reasons:

1) There are countless other astonishing advantages of activity.

Practicing ought not to be finished as discipline for eating an additional cut of cake or to "procure" your food. We believe you should practice given all the great physical and psychological well-being benefits it can bring you!

The blend of activity and good dieting frequently brings about taking less debilitated time from work. The individuals who work out and eat right have a more grounded invulnerable framework and are bound to have the option to fend off diseases. A more grounded resistant framework implies you will not need to go home after the day's work and chance of losing pay. It likewise implies that when you're not working, you will be adequately solid to take part in the exercises you appreciate.

Another advantage is that appropriate sustenance and exercise might diminish your probability of being determined to have specific ailments like osteoporosis, Type 2 diabetes, hypertension, stroke, and coronary illness. In those all around analyzed, practice and good dieting might assist with controlling the side effects and make the disease less meddling in your life.

Stress Reduction

Stress is something everybody experiences, except many individuals, who have found diet and exercise make it simpler to make due. Indeed, even something really basic enough to free a ton of stress you experience consistently. By eating adjusted dinners and working out, you are bound to have a similar degree of energy the entire day, consistently. If your eating routine or potentially practice is irregular, your energy levels will presumably drop at specific times, frequently when you want the energy the most.

A portion of those inconceivable advantages include:

1) Better pressure the executives and decreased hazard of sorrow,More grounded bones and muscles,Decreased hazard of certain malignant growths,Decreased chance of heart sicknesses,Stable glucose and insulin levels,Further developed insight,Better rest,Better sexual wellbeing,

Longer life.

The rundown goes on, however, on top of this large number of advantages, exercise can assist you with doing everything you love throughout everyday life. Whether it's playing with your children and grandchildren, venturing to the far corners of the planet, hitting the dance floor with your mate, climbing on the ends of the week, strolling up the steps to your

#1 café, or going through midday in the kitchen baking, you want to have the actual strength and perseverance to do these things forever.

Making exercise a piece of your routine is fundamental for carrying on with a solid and satisfying life!

2) Calories aren't just scorched in the exercise center

Taking into account food and exercise as an exchange is tricky because actually, the rec center is certainly not a compelling method for consuming calories. In the plan of things, your body consumes your everyday exercises more than in an hour meeting in the rec center. This is called Non-Exercise Activity Thermogenesis (NEAT).

Making development a piece of your life, through activities like a standing work area, customary strolls, using the stairwell, going shopping for food as opposed to requesting on the web, and tossing in an irregular 10 air squats consistently, is a far greater value for your money than zeroing in just on practice in the exercise center.

However, this doesn't mean avoiding your exercise center meetings! Recall every one of the advantages we recorded previously.

3) It makes an undesirable relationship between food and exercise

Taking into account food and exercise as an immediate exchange can make an undesirable outlook. Rather than practicing cherishing your body and eating to sustain it, the relationship can be handed into a mechanical calorie over, calories out.

Over the long haul, this can be twisting into prohibitive dietary patterns and fanatical working out. However, once more, the connection between what you eat and your exercise center meetings are by all accounts not the only factors that can impact body piece changes, and body synthesis changes are not by any means the only motivations to eat and move.

4) It overlooks different variables that impact weight reduction

Alongside NEAT, there are such countless different variables that assume a part in weight reduction past activity. Rest, hydration, processing, food quality, chemicals, stress, climate, and circadian beat all have their part to play in digestion, losing fat, and acquiring muscle.

Forgetting to address these variables can forestall weight reduction, yet in addition, have long haul wellbeing results. It's vital to think about food and exercise.

Eating food is calories going in. Practicing is calories going out. In any case, these activities are far beyond this misrepresented exchange.

Eat and move for smartness, to improve your everyday capability, and to assist your everyday capability, and to assist you with carrying on with a satisfied life. Not simply to consume and consume calories.

Chapter 4

Staying Active While Working Out

Although many individuals view the practice as a method for shedding pounds, it assumes a vital part in the prosperity of the body past weight reduction. Research firmly upholds its advantages across a scope of physical and emotional wellness conditions for individuals, all things considered. Nonetheless, bustling ways of life and a climate that energizes being stationary for a long time of the day (driving house to house, sitting at an office work area, unwinding for the night before a TV) have prompted practice positioning low as fundamentally important for some individuals.

Kinds of Exercise

A wide range of activities offers medical advantages.

Performing various sorts of activities can grow the scope of advantages much further. Yet, it is vital to recall that some activity is superior to none and that almost everybody can take part in some type of activity securely.

Vigorous/Cardiovascular active work. These are exercises that are adequately extraordinary and performed to the point of keeping up with or working on one's heart and lung wellness. Models: strolling, running, moving, bicycling, b-ball, soccer, swimming,muscle-reinforcing action. This might be alluded to as obstruction preparing. These exercises keep up with or increment muscle strength, perseverance, and power. Models: weight machines, freeloads, obstruction, flexible groups, Pilates, everyday exercises of living (lifting kids, conveying food or clothing, climbing steps).

Adaptability preparing. This might be alluded to as extending. It extends or utilizes a skeletal muscle to the mark of pressure, and holds for a few seconds to expand flexibility and scope of movement around a joint. Further developing adaptability can improve the general actual exhibition of different sorts of activity. Models: dynamic stretches performed with development (yoga, jujitsu), static stretches without development (holding a posture for a few seconds or longer), detached extending (utilizing an outer power like a lash or wall to hold a prolonged posture), and dynamic extending (holding a posture without an outside force)

Balance preparing. These exercises are planned to lose one's equilibrium to further develop body control and dependability. They can assist with forestalling falls and different wounds. Models: remaining on one foot, strolling impact point to toe in an entirely straight line, remaining on an equilibrium or wobble board

Proportions of Exercise Intensity

Albeit simply moving more and sitting less offers medical advantages, how much energy you use while practicing can expand those medical advantages further. This is alluded to as an energy force.

Normal exercise wounds include:

Strained or pulled muscles, Lower leg sprain, Knee strain,Aggravated ligaments or tendons,Rotator sleeve (shoulder) injury,Abuse wounds brought about by monotonous developments utilizing fundamentally one piece of the body

In extremely uncommon cases, vivacious active work might prompt a cardiovascular failure or unexpected demise. Dynamic individuals have a lower chance of serious or deadly heart issues than dormant individuals.

Normal stumbles:

Not conversing with your PCP first. Assuming that you are new to the practice or have ailments, let your PCP in on what sort of activity you'll begin. They can survey the organization to guarantee it is protected with a particular ailment.

Doing an excess too early. This is exceptionally normal as individuals might be profoundly energetic while beginning another activity program. In any case, driving your body to move with an excess of force can be jolting to the heart, muscles, and joints that might need strength from idleness. This frequently prompts injury. Regardless of whether beginning gradually feels excessively simple, plan to steadily advance activity.

Begin with light to direct power developments for a more limited measure of time, and proceed with this for half a month. As you foster strength and endurance, you can add minutes and higher-force developments at regular intervals.

Leaving out the warm-up and chill off. A warm-up before

practicing incorporates light developments that start the progression of blood and releasing of muscles and joints. A model would be 5-10 minutes of walking set up, doing arm circles, and neck rolls. In the wake of working out, the cool-down is essential to dial back the body and pulse consistently, as an unexpected stop in development can obstruct the bloodstream to the cerebrum and cause unsteadiness or dizziness.

A cool-down could be easing back the speed of anything that exercise is being performed for 10 minutes (if running, change to a walk; if on an exercise bike, discharge any pressure on the opposition handle and hawk more slowly).

The cool-down time frame may likewise incorporate stretches that are best when the muscles are warmed from working out; extends help to protract muscles that will safeguard against wounds. A cool-down with extending can likewise diminish muscle touchiness the next day.

www.ingramcontent.com/pod-product-compliance
Lightning Source LLC
LaVergne TN
LVHW020534160826
845677LV00015B/4049

9798849464077